INTRODUCTION

Reversing Type 2 Diabetes Through Diet:

Type 2 diabetes, once considered a lifelong condition requiring strict management, is now increasingly

UNDERSTANDING TYPE 2 DIABETES DIET

A Guide to prediabetes and type 2 diabetes diet cookbook to balance your blood sugar and boost your energy

DR TEMMY JOHN

TABLE OF CONTENT

recognized as a condition that can be reversed or significantly improved through lifestyle changes, particularly dietary modifications. This shift in understanding has sparked hope and motivation for millions of individuals diagnosed with this metabolic disorder.

Type 2 diabetes is characterized by insulin resistance and impaired glucose metabolism, leading to elevated blood sugar levels. Traditionally, treatment has focused on medications to control blood sugar, along with dietary recommendations aimed at managing symptoms. However, recent research has highlighted the profound impact that diet can have on the progression and even reversal of this condition.

In this book, we delve into the transformative power of nutrition in the context of type 2 diabetes management. We explore the fundamental principles of a diabetes-reversing diet, backed by scientific evidence and real-life success stories. By understanding the role of specific nutrients, the glycemic impact of foods, and the importance of meal timing and portion control, readers will gain insight into how dietary choices can influence blood sugar regulation and overall health.

The journey to reversing type 2 diabetes through diet is not just about restriction; it's about empowerment and abundance. Through delicious recipes, practical meal plans, and lifestyle strategies, we aim to equip readers with the tools they need to take control of their health and transform their relationship with food.

Whether you've recently been diagnosed with type 2 diabetes, have been managing the condition for years, or simply want to adopt a healthier lifestyle to prevent its onset, this book is your comprehensive guide to embracing dietary changes that can lead to lasting wellness and vitality. Together, let's embark on a journey to reverse type 2 diabetes and reclaim the joy of healthy living.

- Understanding Type 2 Diabetes

Type 2 diabetes is a chronic condition characterized by elevated blood sugar levels resulting from either the body's inability to produce enough insulin or its ineffective use of insulin. Insulin is a hormone produced by the pancreas that regulates glucose (sugar) uptake into cells for energy use. In Type 2 diabetes, cells become resistant to insulin's action, leading to a buildup of glucose in the bloodstream.

Understanding Type 2 diabetes involves recognizing its risk factors, such as obesity, sedentary lifestyle, genetics, and age. While genetics play a role, lifestyle choices significantly influence its development and progression. Poor dietary habits, high sugar intake, and lack of physical activity contribute to insulin resistance and obesity, both central to Type 2 diabetes.

Increased thirst, frequent urination, exhaustion, impaired vision, and sluggish wound healing are all signs of Type 2 diabetes. However, the condition may remain asymptomatic for years, leading to complications such as cardiovascular disease, kidney failure, and nerve damage if left untreated

Managing Type 2 diabetes involves lifestyle modifications such as adopting a healthy diet, regular exercise, weight management, and monitoring blood sugar levels. Medications like oral hypoglycemic agents or insulin therapy may also be prescribed to control blood sugar levels.

Educating individuals about the risk factors, symptoms, and management strategies of Type 2 diabetes is crucial in preventing its onset and reducing its impact on health and quality of life. Early diagnosis, coupled with effective management, can help individuals with Type 2 diabetes lead fulfilling lives while minimizing complications.

- **What is Type 2 Diabetes?**

Chronic metabolic disease known as type 2 diabetes is typified by high blood glucose (sugar) levels. Unlike Type 1 diabetes, where the body fails to produce insulin, or produces very little, Type 2 diabetes involves insulin resistance or the body's inability to use insulin effectively. Insulin, produced by the pancreas, is a hormone that helps regulate blood sugar levels by facilitating the uptake of glucose into cells for energy.

In Type 2 diabetes, cells become resistant to insulin's action, leading to a buildup of glucose in the bloodstream. This results in high blood sugar levels, which, if left uncontrolled, can cause serious health complications over time.

Risk factors for Type 2 diabetes include obesity, physical inactivity, poor dietary habits (such as high consumption of processed foods and sugary beverages), genetics, and age (particularly for those over 45 years old). While genetics plays a role, lifestyle factors significantly contribute to the development and progression of Type 2 diabetes.

Increased thirst, frequent urination, weariness, hazy vision, sluggish wound healing, and recurring infections are some of the symptoms of type 2 diabetes. However, the condition can also be asymptomatic for years, making early detection through regular screenings important.

Management of Type 2 diabetes typically involves lifestyle modifications such as adopting a healthy diet, engaging in regular physical activity, maintaining a healthy weight, monitoring blood sugar levels, and, in some cases, taking medications or insulin therapy as prescribed by healthcare professionals. Effective management can help prevent complications and improve overall quality of life for individuals living with Type 2 diabetes.

- Causes and Risk Factors

Type 2 diabetes is influenced by a combination of genetic, lifestyle, and environmental factors. While the exact causes are not fully understood, several factors contribute to the development of the condition:

1. Genetics: Family history plays a significant role in Type 2 diabetes risk. Having a close relative, such as a parent or sibling, with the condition increases one's likelihood of developing it.

2. Insulin Resistance: Insulin resistance occurs when cells in the body become less responsive to insulin, impairing glucose uptake. Over time, the pancreas compensates by producing more insulin, but eventually, it may not keep up with demand, leading to high blood sugar levels.

3. Obesity: Excess body weight, particularly abdominal fat, increases the risk of insulin resistance and Type 2 diabetes. Adipose tissue releases chemicals that can interfere with insulin's action, contributing to elevated blood sugar levels.

4. Physical Inactivity: Lack of regular physical activity is associated with an increased risk of Type 2 diabetes. Exercise helps improve insulin sensitivity, promotes weight management, and contributes to overall metabolic health.

5. Unhealthy Diet: Consuming a diet high in processed foods, refined carbohydrates, sugars, and saturated fats can contribute to obesity, insulin resistance, and elevated blood sugar levels. Conversely, a diet rich in fruits, vegetables, whole grains, and lean proteins can lower the risk of Type 2 diabetes.

6. Age: While Type 2 diabetes can occur at any age, the risk increases with age, especially after 45 years old. This is partly due to decreased physical activity, muscle mass, and changes in hormone levels associated with aging.

7. Ethnicity: Certain ethnic groups, including African Americans, Hispanic/Latino Americans, Native Americans, and Asian Americans, have a higher predisposition to developing Type 2 diabetes compared to others.

8. **Gestational Diabetes: Women who experience gestational diabetes during pregnancy have an increased risk of developing Type 2 diabetes later in life.

Understanding these causes and risk factors is crucial for prevention efforts and early intervention to reduce the incidence and impact of Type 2 diabetes on individuals and communities. Adopting a healthy lifestyle, including regular physical activity, a balanced diet, weight management, and routine screenings, can help mitigate these risk factors and prevent or delay the onset of Type 2 diabetes.

- Diet is Important for Managing Diabetes Type 2

Diet plays a crucial role in managing Type 2 diabetes as it directly impacts blood sugar levels, weight management, and overall health. Here are several key reasons why diet is important in managing Type 2 diabetes:

1. Blood Sugar Control: The foods we eat directly affect blood sugar levels. Carbohydrates, in particular, have the most significant impact on blood glucose levels. Managing carbohydrate intake, choosing complex carbohydrates with a lower glycemic index, and balancing carbohydrate consumption with protein and healthy fats can help regulate blood sugar levels throughout the day.

2. Weight Management: Excess body weight, especially abdominal fat, is a significant risk factor for Type 2 diabetes and can exacerbate insulin resistance. A healthy diet can aid in weight management by controlling calorie intake, promoting satiety, and providing essential nutrients. Emphasizing whole, nutrient-dense

foods such as fruits, vegetables, lean proteins, and whole grains while limiting processed foods, sugary beverages, and high-calorie snacks can support weight loss or weight maintenance goals.

3. Improving Insulin Sensitivity: Certain dietary patterns, such as the Mediterranean diet or the Dietary Approaches to Stop Hypertension (DASH) diet, have been shown to improve insulin sensitivity and reduce the risk of Type 2 diabetes complications. These diets emphasize whole foods, including fruits, vegetables, whole grains, nuts, seeds, and healthy fats, while limiting refined carbohydrates, added sugars, and saturated fats.

4. Preventing Complications: Well-managed blood sugar levels can help prevent or delay the onset of diabetes-related complications such as cardiovascular disease, neuropathy, kidney disease, and eye problems. A balanced diet that supports blood sugar control and overall health can contribute to reducing the risk of these complications.

5. Enhancing Overall Health: A healthy diet rich in nutrients, antioxidants, and fiber can boost immune function, reduce inflammation, and support cardiovascular health, all of which are important for individuals with Type 2 diabetes who may be at higher risk of other chronic conditions.

In summary, adopting a balanced, nutritious diet tailored to individual needs and preferences is essential for managing Type 2 diabetes effectively. Working with healthcare professionals, such as registered dietitians or nutritionists, can provide personalized guidance and support to develop dietary strategies that promote blood sugar control, weight management, and overall well-being.

Chapter 1

Foundation of a Diabetes-Friendly Diet

The foundation of a diabetes-friendly diet is built on principles that help regulate blood sugar levels, promote weight management, and support overall health. Here are the key components:

1. Carbohydrate Management: Focus on consuming carbohydrates with a low glycemic index (GI) to minimize blood sugar spikes. Choose whole grains like quinoa, brown rice, and barley, as well as legumes, fruits, and vegetables, which provide fiber and essential nutrients while releasing glucose more slowly into the bloodstream.

2. Portion Control: Be mindful of portion sizes to manage carbohydrate intake and prevent overeating, which can lead to blood sugar fluctuations and weight gain. Using measuring

cups, food scales, or visual cues can help gauge appropriate portion sizes.

3. Balanced Meals: Try to have meals that are well-balanced, with a mix of healthy fats, protein, and carbs. Protein-rich foods like lean meats, poultry, fish, tofu, beans, and low-fat dairy help stabilize blood sugar levels and promote satiety, while healthy fats from sources like avocados, nuts, seeds, and olive oil provide sustained energy.

4. Fiber-Rich Foods: Incorporate fiber-rich foods such as fruits, vegetables, whole grains, legumes, and nuts into your diet. Fiber helps slow down the absorption of sugar, promotes digestive health, and contributes to feeling full and satisfied after meals.

5. Limit Added Sugars and Refined Carbohydrates: Minimize consumption of sugary beverages, sweets, desserts, and processed foods high in added sugars and refined carbohydrates. These foods can cause rapid spikes in blood sugar levels and contribute to weight gain.

6. Healthy Cooking Methods: Opt for cooking methods that involve minimal added fats and oils, such as baking, grilling, steaming, and broiling. Use herbs, spices, and citrus juices to enhance flavor without relying on salt or sugar.

7. Regular Meal Timing: Maintain consistent meal times and spacing throughout the day to help stabilize blood sugar levels and prevent large fluctuations. Aim for three balanced

meals and healthy snacks as needed to avoid prolonged periods of hunger.

8. Hydration: Make sure you drink lots of water all day long to stay hydrated. Limit sugary beverages and opt for water, herbal teas, or sparkling water with no added sugars.

9. Individualized Approach: Work with a registered dietitian or healthcare professional to develop a personalized meal plan that takes into account your individual preferences, cultural background, lifestyle, and nutritional needs.

By following these foundational principles, individuals with diabetes can create a sustainable and enjoyable eating pattern that supports blood sugar control, weight management, and overall well-being. Regular monitoring of blood sugar levels and adjustments to dietary choices may be necessary to achieve optimal health outcomes.

- The Role of Carbohydrates, Proteins, and Fats

Carbohydrates, proteins, and fats all play crucial roles in a diabetes-friendly diet, affecting blood sugar levels, energy levels, and overall health.

1. Carbohydrates: Carbohydrates are the body's primary source of energy and have the most significant impact on blood sugar levels. Managing carbohydrate intake is essential for individuals with diabetes to prevent

blood sugar spikes. Carbohydrates are found in foods such as grains, fruits, vegetables, dairy products, and sweets. Choosing complex carbohydrates with a low glycemic index (GI), such as whole grains, legumes, and non-starchy vegetables, can help regulate blood sugar levels more effectively than simple carbohydrates like refined grains and sugary snacks. Portion control and pairing carbohydrates with protein and healthy fats can also help mitigate their impact on blood sugar.

2. Proteins: Protein-rich foods play a vital role in stabilizing blood sugar levels, promoting satiety, and supporting muscle health. Including lean sources of protein such as poultry, fish, tofu, legumes, and low-fat dairy in meals and snacks can help regulate blood sugar and prevent overeating. Protein also aids in repairing and building tissues, making it essential for overall health and well-being.

3. Fats: Healthy fats are an important component of a diabetes-friendly diet, providing sustained energy and supporting heart health. Avocados, almonds, seeds, olive oil, and fatty fish like trout and salmon are good sources of healthful fats. These fats contribute to more stable blood sugar levels by delaying the absorption of carbohydrates. Additionally, omega-3 fatty acids found in fatty fish have anti-inflammatory properties and may reduce the risk of cardiovascular complications associated with diabetes. However, portion control is

important as fats are calorie-dense, and excessive intake can contribute to weight gain.

In summary, balancing carbohydrates, proteins, and fats is key to managing blood sugar levels and promoting overall health in individuals with diabetes. A diabetes-friendly diet should emphasize complex carbohydrates with a low glycemic index, lean sources of protein, and healthy fats while limiting refined carbohydrates, added sugars, and saturated fats. Consulting with a registered dietitian or healthcare professional can provide personalized guidance and support in creating a nutritious and sustainable meal plan tailored to individual needs and preferences.

- Understanding Glycemic Index and Glycemic Load

The Glycemic Index (GI) and Glycemic Load (GL) are two important concepts related to the impact of food on blood sugar levels. Understanding these concepts can help individuals, especially those with diabetes or those who want to manage their blood sugar levels, make informed dietary choices.

Carbohydrates are ranked from 0 to 100 on the Glycemic Index (GI) according to how quickly they boost blood sugar levels after eating. Pure glucose is used as the reference point and is given a GI of 100. Other carbohydrates are compared to glucose and given a GI value accordingly. A high GI indicates a rapid increase in blood sugar, while a low GI indicates a gradual increase.

Foods with a high GI (above 70) include white bread, sugary drinks, and refined grains, while foods with a low GI (below 55) include whole grains, non-starchy vegetables, and most fruits.

Glycemic Load (GL) takes into account the amount of carbohydrates consumed, in addition to the GI. It is calculated by multiplying the GI of a food by the amount of carbohydrates in a serving, divided by 100. GL provides a more accurate representation of the impact of a food on blood sugar levels, as it considers both the quality and quantity of carbohydrates.

A low GL (below 10) is generally considered desirable, as it indicates a minimal impact on blood sugar levels. By understanding the GI and GL of different foods, individuals can make informed choices to manage their blood sugar levels and maintain overall health. This is particularly important for individuals with diabetes, as it can help them manage their condition and reduce the risk of complications.

- Importance of Fiber and Micronutrients

Fiber and micronutrients are essential components of a healthy diet, playing critical roles in maintaining overall well-being and preventing chronic diseases.

Fiber, found in whole grains, fruits, vegetables, and legumes, offers numerous benefits:

- Encourages healthy blood sugar levels and weight management
- Supports regular bowel movements and digestive health
- Lowers cholesterol levels and reduces cardiovascular risk
- Feeds beneficial gut bacteria, boosting the immune system

Micronutrients, such as vitamins and minerals, are essential for a number of body processes.

- Calcium and vitamin D for strong bones
- Iron for healthy red blood cells
- Vitamin C for immune function and collagen production
- Omega-3 fatty acids to support brain and cardiac health

Consuming enough fiber and micronutrients can be beneficial.

- Lower the chance of developing long-term conditions like diabetes, heart disease, and some types of cancer
- Support healthy growth and development in children and adolescents

- Maintain healthy skin, hair, and nails
- Boost energy levels and mental clarity

Unfortunately, many individuals fall short of the recommended daily intake of fiber and micronutrients, increasing their risk of deficiency-related health issues. To reap the benefits, focus on consuming a balanced diet rich in whole, unprocessed foods, and consider supplements if necessary. Prioritizing fiber and micronutrient intake is a simple yet powerful step towards achieving optimal health and well-being.

- Portion Control and Meal Timing

Portion control and meal timing are crucial aspects of a healthy diet, playing a significant role in maintaining optimal weight, regulating blood sugar levels, and promoting overall well-being.

Portion control refers to the amount of food consumed in one sitting. Eating large portions can lead to consuming more calories, sugar, and unhealthy fats than needed, increasing the risk of chronic diseases like obesity, diabetes, and heart disease. Practicing portion control by:
- Eating appropriate serving sizes
- Avoiding second helpings
- Choosing smaller plates

can help:
- Reduce overall calorie intake
- Manage hunger and satiety cues

- Develop healthy eating habits

Meal timing, on the other hand, refers to the frequency and timing of meals throughout the day. Eating regular, balanced meals can help:
- Regulate blood sugar levels
- Boost metabolism
- Support energy levels and focus

Aim for:
- Three main courses plus one or two snacks
- Eating within an hour of waking up and at least two hours before bedtime
- Incorporating protein and healthy fats with each meal

By practicing portion control and mindful meal timing, individuals can:
- Improve nutrient absorption and digestion
- Support weight management and overall health
- Reduce the risk of chronic diseases

Remember, developing healthy habits takes time and practice, but the benefits to overall well-being are worth the effort.

Chapter 2:

Essential Ingredients for Diabetes Wellness

Living with diabetes requires a careful balance of nutrition, exercise, and lifestyle habits to manage blood sugar levels and promote overall well-being. While there is no single "diabetes diet," incorporating essential ingredients into your meals can help support diabetes wellness. These ingredients are rich in nutrients, fiber, and antioxidants, which can help regulate blood sugar, improve insulin sensitivity, and reduce inflammation.

Leafy greens like spinach, kale, and collard greens are packed with antioxidants and fiber, making them an excellent addition to your diet. Berries, such as blueberries, raspberries, and strawberries, are high in antioxidants and fiber, and can be enjoyed as a snack or added to oatmeal or yogurt.

Nuts and seeds like almonds, chia seeds, and flaxseeds are rich in healthy fats and protein, supporting heart health and satiety. Fatty fish like salmon, tuna, and mackerel are high in omega-3 fatty acids, which can help reduce inflammation and improve heart health.

Sweet potatoes are rich in fiber and antioxidants, making them a great alternative to white potatoes. Avocados are high in healthy fats and fiber, supporting heart health and satiety. Legumes like lentils, chickpeas, and black beans are rich in protein and fiber, making them an excellent source of plant-based protein.

Whole grains like brown rice, quinoa, and whole wheat provide fiber and antioxidants, supporting digestive health and satiety. Herbs and spices like turmeric, cinnamon, and ginger have anti-inflammatory properties, which can help reduce inflammation and improve insulin sensitivity.

Fermented foods like yogurt, kimchi, and sauerkraut support gut health, which is essential for immune function and overall well-being. Tea, especially green tea, is rich in antioxidants and can help reduce inflammation and improve insulin sensitivity. Dark chocolate, with at least 70% cocoa content, is rich in antioxidants and can be enjoyed in moderation as a sweet treat.

Incorporating these essential ingredients into your diet can help support diabetes wellness by regulating blood sugar levels, improving insulin sensitivity, and reducing inflammation. Remember to consult with a healthcare professional or registered dietitian for personalized dietary advice.

- Selecting Healthy Carbohydrates

Selecting healthy carbohydrates is crucial for maintaining a balanced diet and managing blood sugar levels.

Here are some tips for choosing healthy carbohydrates:

1. Focus on whole, unprocessed foods:
   - Whole grains (brown rice, quinoa, whole wheat)
   - Vegetables (leafy greens, broccoli, bell peppers)
   - Fruits (apples, berries, citrus fruits)

- Legumes (lentils, chickpeas, black beans)
2. Choose complex carbohydrates:
   - Whole grains contain fiber, vitamins, and minerals
   - Vegetables and fruits are rich in fiber, antioxidants, and phytochemicals
3. Limit refined and processed carbohydrates:
   - Sugary drinks, baked items, and white bread
   - Refined grains (white rice, pasta, sugary cereals)
4. Be mindful of portion sizes:
   - Eat appropriate serving sizes to manage carbohydrate intake
5. Consider the glycemic index (GI):
   - Choose low-GI foods (whole grains, vegetables, fruits) to manage blood sugar levels

Remember, a balanced diet with a variety of whole, unprocessed foods provides the necessary carbohydrates for energy and overall healthSee a medical practitioner or qualified dietician for individualized dietary guidance.

- Lean Proteins for Sustained Energy

Lean proteins are an essential part of a healthy diet, providing sustained energy and supporting overall well-being. Here are some benefits and examples of lean proteins:

Benefits:
- Provides sustained energy

- Supports muscle growth and maintenance
- Helps with weight management
- Supports overall health and well-being

Examples:
- Poultry: chicken, turkey, duck
- Fish: salmon, tuna, tilapia, cod
- Legumes: kidney beans, black beans, chickpeas, and lentils
- Nuts and seeds: almonds, chia seeds, hemp seeds
- Whole grains: quinoa, farro, bulgur
- Dairy: cottage cheese, Greek yogurt, and low-fat milk
- Meat: lean beef, pork tenderloin, venison

Tips:
- Choose grass-fed, hormone-free, and organic options when possible
- Vary your protein sources to ensure you're getting all essential amino acids
- The daily goal should be 0.8–1 grams of protein per pound of body weight.
- Combine protein with complex carbohydrates for sustained energy

Incorporating lean proteins into your diet can help support sustained energy, muscle growth, and overall health. Remember to choose a variety of protein sources and combine them with complex carbohydrates for optimal energy and well-being.

- Heart-Healthy Fats and Oils

Heart-healthy fats and oils are essential for maintaining overall health and well-being. Here are some examples and benefits:

Examples:
- Monounsaturated fats:
    - Avocados
    - Olive oil
    - Nuts (almonds, cashews, pecans)
    - Seeds (pumpkin, sunflower)
- Polyunsaturated fats:
    - Fatty fish (salmon, tuna, mackerel)
    - Nuts (walnuts, flaxseeds, chia seeds)
    - Seeds (hemp, canola)
- Omega-3 fatty acids:
    - Fatty fish (salmon, sardines, anchovies)
    - Flaxseeds
    - Chia seeds
    - Walnuts

Benefits:
- Reduce LDL ("bad") cholesterol and total cholesterol.
- Increase HDL ("good") cholesterol
- Reduce risk of heart disease and stroke
- Support brain function and development
- Aid in absorption of vitamins and minerals

Tips:
- Use olive oil for cooking and dressing salads
- Snack on nuts and seeds
- Incorporate fatty fish into your diet
- Restrict your intake of red meat, full-fat dairy products, and processed snacks to a minimum.
- Read labels and choose products with healthy fats and oils

Remember, a balanced diet with a variety of whole foods provides the necessary heart-healthy fats and oils for optimal well-being. For individualized nutrition recommendations, speak with a licensed dietitian or other healthcare provider.

- Incorporating Fiber-Rich Foods

Including foods high in fiber in your diet can provide a number of health advantages, such as:
- Promoting regular bowel movements and preventing constipation
- Supporting healthy blood sugar levels
- Lowering cholesterol levels and reducing the risk of heart disease
- Aiding in weight management
- Supporting healthy gut bacteria

Here are some high-fiber foods to include in your diet:
- Fruits:
  - Berries (raspberries, strawberries, blueberries)
  - Apples
  - Bananas
  - Oranges
- Vegetables:
  - Leafy greens (broccoli, spinach, kale)
  - Carrots
  - Peas
  - Sweet potatoes
- Legumes:
  - Lentils

- Chickpeas
  - Black beans
  - Kidney beans
- Whole grains:
  - Brown rice
  - Quinoa
  - Whole wheat bread
  - Whole grain pasta
- Nuts and seeds:
  - Almonds
  - Chia seeds
  - Flaxseeds
  - Pumpkin seeds

Tips for increasing fiber intake:

- Start with small amounts and gradually increase fiber intake to allow your gut to adjust
- Eat a variety of fiber-rich foods to ensure you're getting a range of fiber types
- Incorporate fiber-rich foods into your meals and snacks
- To aid in the passage of fiber through your digestive tract, drink lots of water.

Aim to consume 25-30 grams of fiber per day for optimal health benefits. If you have specific dietary needs or restrictions, consult a healthcare professional or registered dietitian for personalized guidance.

- Herbs, Spices, and Flavor Enhancers

Herbs, spices, and flavor enhancers are a great way to add flavor and depth to your cooking without adding extra salt, sugar, or unhealthy fats. Herbs are the leaves, stems, or flowers of plants used for flavoring, while spices are the seeds, bark, roots, or fruit of plants. Flavor enhancers are ingredients that enhance the natural flavor of food without adding extra salt or sugar.

Using herbs, spices, and flavor enhancers can have numerous health benefits. For example, turmeric contains curcumin, which has anti-inflammatory properties, while ginger has natural anti-inflammatory compounds like gingerol and shogaol. Cinnamon has been shown to lower blood sugar levels and improve insulin sensitivity.

Some popular herbs and spices include:
- Basil
- Oregano
- Thyme
- Cumin
- Coriander
- Paprika
- Garam masala
- Chili powder
- Cinnamon
- Ginger
- Turmeric

Flavor enhancers like lemon juice, vinegar, and umami-rich ingredients like mushrooms, soy sauce, and miso paste can add depth and richness to dishes without added salt or sugar.

When using herbs, spices, and flavor enhancers, remember:
- Start with modest quantities and taste as needed

- Combine different herbs and spices to create unique flavor profiles
- Use fresh herbs whenever possible
- Store spices and herbs in a cool, dark place to preserve flavor and aroma
- Experiment with different flavor enhancers to find what works best for you

By incorporating herbs, spices, and flavor enhancers into your cooking, you can create delicious, healthy, and flavorful meals that will tantalize your taste buds and support your overall well-being.

Chapter 3

Planning Balanced Meals

Planning balanced meals is an essential aspect of maintaining a healthy diet and lifestyle. A balanced meal provides the body with the necessary nutrients, vitamins, and minerals to function properly, and can help prevent chronic diseases such as heart disease, diabetes, and certain cancers. In this article, we will explore the key components of a balanced meal and provide tips on how to plan healthy meals for yourself and your family.

Key Components of a Balanced Meal:

1. Protein: Includes foods such as lean meats, poultry, fish, eggs, dairy products, legumes, and nuts. Building

and mending muscles, organs, and tissues require protein.

2. Whole Grains: Includes foods such as brown rice, quinoa, whole wheat bread, whole grain pasta, and oats. Whole grains provide fiber, vitamins, and minerals.

3. Vegetables: Includes a variety of colorful vegetables such as leafy greens, broccoli, bell peppers, carrots, and tomatoes. Vegetables provide vitamins, minerals, and antioxidants.

4. Fruits: Includes a variety of fruits such as apples, bananas, berries, and citrus fruits. Fruits provide vitamins, minerals, and antioxidants.

5. Healthy Fats: Includes foods such as nuts, seeds, avocado, and olive oil. Healthy fats provide energy and support heart health.

Tips for Planning Balanced Meals:

1. Plan your meals in advance: Take some time each week to plan out your meals for the next few days. This will help you avoid last-minute, unhealthy choices.

2. Shop smart: Make a grocery list based on your meal plan and stick to it. Try to shop the perimeter of the grocery store, where the fresh produce, meats, and dairy products are typically located.

3. Prepare meals at home: This gives you more control over the components and serving sizes of your meals. Try to prepare dinner most nights of the week at home.

4. Include a variety of colors: Aim to include a variety of colorful fruits and

vegetables in your meals to ensure you are getting a range of vitamins and minerals.

5. Watch portion sizes: Pay attention to the serving sizes of your meals and snacks to maintain a healthy weight and prevent chronic diseases.

6. Make leftovers work for you: Cook in bulk and use leftovers for future meals to save time and reduce food waste.

7. Involve the whole family: Encourage everyone in the household to get involved in meal planning and cooking. This can help teach children important skills and promote healthy eating habits.

In conclusion, planning balanced meals is crucial for maintaining a healthy diet and lifestyle. By including a variety of protein, whole grains, vegetables, fruits, and healthy fats in your meals, you can ensure you are providing your body with the necessary nutrients to function properly. Remember to plan your meals in advance, shop smart, cook at home, include a variety of colors, watch portion sizes, make leftovers work for you, and involve the whole family in meal planning and cooking.

- Meal Planning Basics for Diabetes Management

One of the most important parts of managing diabetes is meal planning. To get you started, consider the following fundamentals of meal planning:

1. Diabetes Plate Method: Divide your plate into three parts:
   - Half: Non-starchy vegetables (e.g., broccoli, spinach, green beans)
   - Quarter: Protein (e.g., chicken, fish, beans)
   - Quarter: Carbohydrates (e.g., whole grains, fruits, starchy vegetables)
2. Count Your Carbohydrates: Carbohydrates affect blood sugar levels. Set a daily limit and count carbs at each meal.
3. Eat Regular Meals: Space out meals to maintain stable blood sugar levels.
4. Choose Whole Foods: Focus on whole, unprocessed foods like vegetables, fruits, whole grains, lean proteins, and healthy fats.
5. Incorporate Protein and Healthy Fats: Protein and healthy fats slow down carbohydrate digestion and absorption.
6. Limit Added Sugars and Refined Grains: Avoid foods with added sugars and refined grains, which can raise blood sugar levels.
7. Stay Hydrated: Drink plenty of water throughout the day.
8. Consult a Registered Dietitian or Certified Diabetes Educator: Get personalized meal planning advice and guidance.

Remember, meal planning for diabetes management is individualized, so work with a healthcare professional to develop a plan that suits your needs.

- Building a Balanced Plate

Building a balanced plate is a simple and effective way to ensure you're getting the nutrients your body needs to thrive. A balanced plate is divided into four sections, each containing a different food group. This visual guide helps you portion your food correctly and creates a harmonious balance of nutrients on your plate.

The four sections of a balanced plate are:

1. Protein (30% of the plate)
   - Includes foods like lean meats, poultry, fish, beans, lentils, and dairy products
   - Provides energy and supports muscle growth and repair
2. Vegetables (40% of the plate)
   - Includes a variety of colorful vegetables like leafy greens, bell peppers, carrots, and tomatoes
   - Rich in vitamins, minerals, and antioxidants
3. Whole Grains (20% of the plate)
   - Includes foods like brown rice, quinoa, whole wheat bread, and whole grain pasta
   - Provides fiber, vitamins, and minerals

Building a balanced plate has numerous benefits, including:

- Supports overall health and well-being
- Manages weight and lowers the chance of developing chronic illnesses

- Provides sustained energy throughout the day
- Supports healthy digestion and bowel function
- Helps maintain healthy blood sugar levels

Tips for building a balanced plate:
- Begin with an assortment of vibrant vegetables
- Add a source of protein
- Include a serving of whole grains
- Add a small amount of healthy fats
- Adjust portion sizes based on individual calorie needs
- Ensure that you have a lot of water with your meal.

Remember, building a balanced plate is a flexible guide, and portions can be adjusted based on individual needs. The key is to create a harmonious balance of nutrients on your plate to support overall health and well-being.

- Snack Ideas for Stable Blood Sugar Levels

Maintaining blood sugar levels throughout the day requires eating snacks. Choosing the right snacks can help keep your blood sugar levels stable, preventing spikes and crashes. The following snack suggestions may be useful:

1. Nuts and Seeds: Almonds, cashews, pumpkin seeds, and chia seeds are all great choices. They're high in healthy fats and protein, which slow down the digestion of carbohydrates, preventing a sudden spike in blood sugar levels.

2. Fresh Fruits: Fresh fruits like apples, berries, and citrus fruits are rich in fiber, vitamins, and minerals. They're also low in calories and carbohydrates, making them an excellent snack for stable blood sugar levels.

3. Vegetables: Crunchy vegetables like carrots, cucumbers, and bell peppers are low in calories and rich in fiber, vitamins, and minerals. They're also very filling, making them an excellent snack for weight management.

4. Protein-Rich Snacks: Greek yogurt, hard-boiled eggs, and cottage cheese are all high in protein, which slows down the digestion of carbohydrates, preventing a sudden spike in blood sugar levels.

5. Whole Grain Crackers: Whole grain crackers are rich in fiber, vitamins, and minerals. They're also low in calories and carbohydrates, making them an excellent snack for stable blood sugar levels. You can top them with avocado, peanut butter, or hummus for added nutrition.

6. Edamame: Edamame is a type of soybean that's high in protein and fiber. It's also low in calories and carbohydrates, making it an excellent snack for stable blood sugar levels.

7. Trail Mix: Trail mix is a combination of nuts, seeds, and dried fruits. It's high in healthy fats and protein, which slow down the digestion of carbohydrates, preventing a sudden spike in blood sugar levels.

8. Popcorn: Air-popped popcorn is a whole grain snack that's low in calories and carbohydrates. It's also high in fiber, vitamins, and minerals, making it an excellent snack for stable blood sugar levels.

9. Smoothies: Smoothies made with Greek yogurt, frozen fruits, and spinach are an excellent snack for stable blood sugar levels. They're high in protein, fiber, and vitamins, and low in calories and carbohydrates.

10. Energy Balls: Energy balls made with oats, nuts, seeds, and dried fruits are an excellent snack for stable blood sugar levels. They're high in healthy fats and protein, which slow down the digestion of carbohydrates, preventing a sudden spike in blood sugar levels.

Remember, portion control is key when it comes to snacking. Choose snacks that are low in calories and carbohydrates, and high in healthy fats and protein. Also, make sure to drink plenty of water throughout the day to stay hydrated.

- Tips for Dining Out and Social Settings

Dining out and social settings can be challenging when managing blood sugar levels, but with some planning and awareness, you can enjoy yourself while keeping your levels under control. Here are some tips:

1. Choose wisely: Opt for restaurants that serve whole, unprocessed foods

and offer healthy options like grilled meats, vegetables, and whole grains.

2. Check the menu ahead: Look up the menu online and plan your meal in advance to ensure healthy options are available.

3. Communicate with your server: Inform your server about your dietary needs and ask for recommendations.

4. Be mindful of portion sizes: Even healthy foods can affect blood sugar levels if consumed in excess.

5. Balance your meal: Pair high-carb foods with protein and healthy fats to slow down digestion and absorption.

6. Don't be afraid to ask for modifications: Request sauces and dressings on the side or ask for a smaller portion of high-carb foods.

7. Stay hydrated: Drink water throughout your meal to help with digestion and prevent dehydration.

8. Be prepared for social situations: If you're attending a buffet or potluck, bring a healthy dish to share and eat before indulging in other options.

9. Don't feel pressured to overindulge: It's okay to say no to foods that may affect your blood sugar levels.

10. Monitor your levels: Check your blood sugar levels before and after eating to understand how different foods affect you.

By following these tips, you can enjoy dining out and social settings while maintaining control over your blood sugar levels. Always put your health first and make well-informed decisions.

Chapter 4:

- Delicious Breakfast Recipes

The most significant meal of the day is breakfast! It's the perfect time to refuel and recharge for the adventures ahead. But, let's be real, mornings can be chaotic, and cooking up a storm in the kitchen might not be on the agenda. That's why we've got you covered with some delicious breakfast recipes that are quick, easy, and packed with flavor!

First up, we have the Crustless Spinach Quiche. This veggie-filled wonder is a game-changer for breakfast lovers. With its creamy eggs, spinach, and feta cheese, it's a nutritious and delicious start to the day. And the best part? It's incredibly easy to make!

Next, we have the Sausage and Egg Casserole. This classic breakfast dish is a crowd-pleaser, and for good reason. With its savory sausage, fluffy eggs, and crispy bread, it's a hearty and satisfying meal that will keep you going all morning long.

But, if you're in a hurry, don't worry! Our Banana Muffins are the perfect on-the-go breakfast solution. Moist, flavorful, and packed with bananas, they're a tasty and convenient way to start your day.

Of course, no breakfast roundup would be complete without some waffles! Our True Belgian Waffles are a classic recipe that yields crispy, golden waffles with a fluffy interior. Top them with fresh fruit, whipped cream, or syrup for a decadent breakfast treat.

If you're looking for something a little sweeter, our Lemon Blueberry Bread is a must-try. This moist and flavorful loaf is packed with lemon zest and juicy blueberries, making it the perfect breakfast or snack.

But, wait, there's more! Our Hash Brown Egg Bake is a simple and easy-to-make breakfast casserole that's perfect for a crowd. With its crispy hash browns, fluffy eggs, and savory sausage, it's a satisfying and delicious meal that's sure to please.

And, finally, we have our Eggs Benedict Casserole. This twist on the classic eggs benedict recipe is a breakfast game-changer. With its poached eggs, crispy bacon, and creamy hollandaise sauce, it's a decadent and delicious start to the day.

So, there you have it - 10 delicious breakfast recipes to start your day off right. We've got you covered whether you're craving something savory or sweet. Have fun in the kitchen!

- Energizing Morning Meals to Start Your Day Right

Here are some energizing morning meals to start your day right

- Bananas*: Bananas are packed with potassium, vitamin B6, and complex carbs, all of which contribute to energy levels.
- Eggs: Eggs are a great source of protein and can provide long-lasting energy.
- Oatmeal: Oatmeal is a great source of carbohydrates and fiber, which can keep you full for longer.
- Cottage Cheese: Cottage cheese is a great source of protein and can keep you satisfied and energized throughout the day.
- Greek Yogurt: Greek yogurt is a great source of probiotics, which can help with digestion and keep you energized throughout the day.
- Avocado: Avocados are a great source of healthy fats, which can provide energy and keep you full for longer.
- Almonds: Almonds are a great source of healthy fats and protein, which can provide energy and keep you full for longer.
- Papaya: Papaya is a great source of vitamin C, which can help with the absorption of iron and provide energy.
- Flaxseed: Flaxseed is a great source of fiber, which can help with digestion and keep you full for longer.
- Chia Seeds: Chia seeds are a great source of fiber and protein, which can provide energy and keep you full for longer.
- Berries: Berries are a great source of antioxidants and vitamin C, which can help with energy and overall health.

- Coconut: Coconut is a great source of healthy fats, which can provide energy and keep you full for longer.
- Tofu: Tofu is a great source of plant-based protein, which can provide energy and keep you full for longer.
- Legumes: Legumes are a great source of plant-based protein, which can provide energy and keep you full for longer.
- Nuts: Nuts are a great source of healthy fats and protein, which can provide energy and keep you full for longer.

- Quick and Easy Breakfast Options

Here are some quick and easy breakfast options
- Sausage & Crescent Roll Breakfast Casserole: This is a savory breakfast recipe that can be prepared the night before to make your morning even easier.
- Ham and Swiss Omelet: This omelet is easy to make and can be prepared for breakfast or dinner.
- Rise and Shine Parfait: This is a sweet and easy-to-make breakfast parfait made with vanilla yogurt, peaches, and blackberries.
- Stuffed Ham & Egg Bread: This is a comforting stuffed bread full of ham, eggs, and cheese.
- Italian Cloud Eggs: These cloud-like eggs are a dreamy breakfast option.

- Breakfast Sweet Potatoes: This is a delicious and fun way to enjoy sweet potatoes for breakfast.
- Fruity Waffle Parfaits: This waffle parfait is a breakfast staple that offers you even more textures and flavors with yogurt and fresh strawberries.
- Waffle Sandwich: This is a breakfast for lunch or dinner option that is easy to make and can be extra crunchy and protein-rich with pistachios or almonds.
- Cornflake-Coated Crispy Bacon: This is a crispy and easy-to-make bacon strip recipe.
- Cream Cheese & Chive Omelet: This is a savory and creamy omelet that is not your ordinary omelet.

- Overnight Oats and Smoothie Recipes

Here are some overnight oats and smoothie recipes

Overnight Oats Recipes

- Basic Overnight Oats: 1/2 cup rolled oats, 1/2 cup milk (dairy or dairy-free), 1/4 cup Greek yogurt (dairy or dairy-free), 1 tablespoon chia seeds, 1 tablespoon maple syrup
- Banana Bread Overnight Oats: 1/2 banana, mashed, 2 tablespoons chopped walnuts, 1/2 teaspoon vanilla extract, 1/2 teaspoon cinnamon, pinch of ground flaxseed
- Spiced Pear Overnight Oats: 1/2 pear, diced, 1 tablespoon chopped pecans, 1/2 teaspoon cinnamon, pinch of nutmeg

- PB&J Overnight Oats: 2 tablespoons raspberry jam or puree, 1 tablespoon peanut butter (or almond butter), 1 teaspoon chopped pistachios
- Pina Colada Overnight Oats: 1/4 cup small diced pineapple, 1 tablespoon shredded coconut, 1/4 teaspoon vanilla extract (use coconut milk in the base recipe)
- Carrot Cake Overnight Oats: 1/4 cup shredded carrot, 1 tablespoon shredded coconut, 1 tablespoon raisins, 1/2 teaspoon vanilla extract, 1/2 teaspoon cinnamon
- Strawberry Protein Overnight Oats: 1/4 cup small diced strawberry, 1 scoop protein powder or collagen powder, 1 tablespoon sliced almonds, 1/2 teaspoon vanilla extract

Overnight Oatmeal Smoothies
- Carrot Cake: 1/2 cup grated carrots, 1/2 cup pineapple, 1/2 tsp. cinnamon, pinch of nutmeg
- Strawberry Cheesecake: 3/4 cup strawberries, 1 tbsp cream cheese, extra sweetener to taste depending on the sweetness of your fruit
- Apple Pie: 3/4 cup cooked apples (or raw), 1 tbsp almond butter, 1/2 tsp. cinnamon
- Chocolate Peanut Butter Banana: 1 chopped banana, 1 tbsp. unsweetened cocoa powder, 1 tbsp. peanut butter. Optional: add 1 cup spinach

Instructions
1. Add all the ingredients into a sealable jar or bowl and give it a stir until combined.

2. Soak it for at least two hours in the refrigerator; however, an eight-hour overnight soak is ideal. This will yield a creamier consistency.

3. Top your overnight oats with your favorite toppings and enjoy!

For smoothies, mix together the oats, yogurt, almond milk, Stevia (or another sweetener), and any spices you are using. Add the flax, chia, and oat seeds and stir. Add your add-ins (fruits, veggies, nut butter, etc.). Keep it covered and refrigerated for a maximum of five days. Blend everything together when you're ready for a smoothie.

- Traditional Breakfast Favorites with a Healthy Twist

Here are some traditional breakfast favorites with a healthy twist

- Old Fashioned Pancakes: Made with whole wheat flour, aluminum-free baking powder, organic raw honey, unsweetened almond milk, coconut oil, and a free-range egg.

- Creamy Lemon Chicken Parmesan: A healthier version of chicken parmesan with a lemony cream sauce made with half-and-half instead of cream and whole-wheat panko breadcrumbs.

- Cauliflower Chicken Fried "Rice": A healthier version of chicken fried rice with cauliflower instead of rice.

- Oven-Fried Fish & Chips: A healthier version of fish and chips with

a crispy cornflake crust and baked instead of fried.
- Chipotle Chicken Quinoa Burrito Bowl: A healthier version of a burrito bowl with quinoa instead of rice and loaded with vegetables.
- BBQ Chicken Tenders: A healthier version of chicken tenders with a light coating of oil and baked instead of fried.
- Shrimp Tacos with Avocado Crema: A healthier version of shrimp tacos with lean shrimp, crunchy vegetables, and avocado crema.
- General Tso's Chicken: A healthier version of General Tso's chicken with reduced-sodium soy sauce and steamed baby bok choy or sautéed spinach and brown rice.

Chapter 5:

Satisfying Lunch Recipes

Here are some satisfying lunch recipes [1] [2].
- Veggie & Hummus Sandwich: A vegetarian sandwich filled with hummus and vegetables.
- Buffalo Chicken Grain Bowl: A nutritious bowl filled with chicken, couscous, and vegetables.
- Chickpea & Roasted Red Pepper Lettuce Wraps: A tangy wrap filled with chickpeas, roasted red peppers, and tahini dressing.

- Chopped Cobb Salad: A single-serving salad filled with chicken, bacon, and honey-mustard vinaigrette.
- 3-Ingredient Creamy Rotisserie Chicken Salad: A chicken salad made with lemon-herb mayonnaise.
- Quesadilla: A Mexican dish filled with cheese (and optional meat or vegetables).
- White Bean and Tuna Salad: A salad filled with tuna, white beans, and olive oil.
- Chickpea Salad Sandwich: A vegetarian sandwich filled with chickpeas and mixed greens.
- Loaded Veggie Sandwich: A sandwich filled with vegetables and avocado.
- Mediterranean Chickpea Salad: A salad filled with chickpeas, artichoke hearts, cucumbers, tomatoes, and olives.

Nutrient-Packed Lunch Ideas for Busy Days

Here are some nutrient-packed lunch ideas for busy days
- Tuna and White Bean Salad: A classic Italian pairing of tuna and cannellini beans makes a simple and satisfying lunch.
- Rice and Bean Freezer Burritos: A budget-friendly recipe that can save you money and sodium.
- Lentil Salad with Feta, Tomatoes, Cucumbers and Olives: A Mediterranean lentil salad with

chopped veggies, feta cheese and a light dressing.
- Black Bean-Quinoa Bowl: A black bean and quinoa bowl with pico de gallo, fresh cilantro and avocado plus an easy hummus dressing to drizzle on top.
- Chopped Cobb Salad: A single-serving recipe for Cobb salad that swaps chicken in for bacon, which makes it a great source of protein for lunch.
- Veggie and Hummus Sandwich: A vegetable and hummus sandwich that makes the perfect heart-healthy vegetarian lunch to go.
- Healthy Turkey Club Sandwich: A sandwich with gluten-free sandwich bun, avocado-based mayonnaise, low-sodium turkey breast, bacon, avocado, lettuce and tomato.
- Turkey Burger and Greens Bento Box: A bento-style lunch box with a cooked turkey burger, broccoli florets, cheese cubes and dressing.
- *Gluten-Free Vegetarian Pasta Salad*: A pasta salad with gluten-free pasta, balsamic vinegar, cannellini beans, tomato, cucumber, red onion, herbs, salt and pepper.
- Healthy Chicken Salad: A chicken salad with cooked shredded chicken, celery, red onion, avocado-based mayo, herbs, lemon juice, salt and pepper.
- Avocado Turkey Roll-Ups: Roll-ups with roasted turkey breast, Dijon mustard and avocado.

- Salads, Wraps, and Sandwiches

Here are some sandwich wrap recipes

- Turkey Strawberry Wrap: Smoked turkey, strawberries, poppy seed dressing, and pecans.
- Cilantro-Lime Shrimp Wrap: Shrimp with cumin, lime juice, cilantro, garlic, oil, salt, and pepper.
- BLT Wrap: Bacon, tomatoes, and mayo.
- Chicken Caesar Wrap: Chicken, bacon, croutons, and caesar dressing.
- Grilled Cheeseburger Wrap: Beef, cheese, and salad.
- Vegan BBQ Jackfruit Wrap: Jackfruit, BBQ sauce, and vegan cheese.
- Ultimate Veggie Wrap: Tomatoes, cucumbers, carrots, sprouts, and cream cheese.
- Creamy Spinach and Feta Cheese Wrap: Spinach, feta, onions, and peppers.
- PF Chang's Chicken Lettuce Wrap: Ground chicken, lettuce, and soy sauce.
- Tuna Wrap: Tuna, yogurt, mustard, walnuts, raisins, parsley, capers, and red pepper flakes.
- Homemade Crunch Wrap Supreme: Beef, cheese, and nacho cheese.
- Easy Pepperoni Pizza Tortilla Wrap: Pepperoni, pizza sauce, and mozzarella.

- Spiced Paneer Wrap: Paneer, tikka masala paste, and veggies.
- Vegan Greek Salad Wrap: Vegan feta, olives, cucumbers, and tomatoes.
- Black Bean and Avocado Wrap: Black beans, avocado, and taco seasoning.
- Mushroom Wrap: Mushrooms, caramelized onions, garlic mayo, and jalapeños.
- Italian Wrap: Ham, salami, chicken, prosciutto, turkey, and vinaigrette.
- Roast Beef and Horseradish Wrap: Roast beef, horseradish sauce, and garlic hummus.
- Cranberry Feta Pinwheel: Cranberries, feta, and cream cheese.
- Smashed Chickpea and Goat Cheese Wrap: Chickpeas, goat cheese, and vegan cream cheese.
- Artichoke Steak Wrap: Artichoke, steak, and lemon.
- Cranberry Turkey Wrap: Cranberries, turkey, cheese, and olives.
- Club Roll-Ups: Chicken, bacon, lettuce, and tomato.
- Beef 'n' Cheese Wrap: Beef, cheese, Caesar dressing, and olives.
- Caesar Chicken Wrap: Chicken, Caesar dressing, and croutons.
- Veggie Brown Rice Wrap: Veggies, brown rice, and salsa.
- Asian Chicken Crunch Wrap: Chicken, veggies, and peanut sauce.
- Turkey Guacamole Wrap: Turkey, avocado, and hot sauce.
- Crunchy Tuna Wrap: Tuna, veggies, and whole grain tortillas.

- Buffalo Tofu Wrap: Tofu, buffalo sauce, and ranch dressing.
- Easy Southwestern Veggie Wrap: Veggies, brown rice, and sour cream.
- Indian Spiced Chickpea Wrap: Chickpeas, Indian spices, and yogurt.
- Mexican Shredded Beef Wrap: Beef, cheese, and salsa.
- Tropical Beef Wrap: Beef, pineapple, and coconut.
- Quick Taco Wrap: Beef, cheese, and salsa.
- Cuban Pork Wrap: Pork, pickles, and mustard.
- Salmon Bean Wrap: Salmon, black beans, and avocado.
- Thai Chicken Wrap: Chicken, broccoli slaw, and peanut sauce.
- Hummus & Veggie Wrap-Up: Hummus, veggies, and whole grain tortillas.
- Chipotle BLT Wrap: Bacon, lettuce, tomato, and chipotle mayo.

- Hearty Soups and Stews

Here are some options for hearty soups and stews [1] [2]:
- Classic Hearty Beef Stew: A classic beef stew recipe that makes the most of each step of the cooking process to end up with a beautiful, rich, and hearty beef stew.
- Creamy Chicken Taco Soup: A slow cooker creamy chicken taco soup reminiscent of the popular dish King Ranch Chicken, in the form of a soup.
- Kale White Bean and Farro Stew: A hearty stew on a classic Italian farro

and bean soup, but with more vegetables.
- Hearty Hamburger Soup: A thick and hearty soup, filling and very good. It is easy and quick to make.
- Hearty Italian Meatball Soup: A hearty Italian meatball soup that you can make with fewer than 10 easy-to-find ingredients.
- Creamy Chicken and Wild Rice Soup: A creamy chicken and wild rice soup perfect for cold rainy days.
- Creamy Chicken Tortellini Soup: A creamy chicken tortellini soup that you can serve with garlic breadsticks.
- Ham and Potato Soup: A delicious ham and potato soup that you can serve with fresh biscuits.
- Brunswick Stew: A classic Brunswick stew that you can make with brisket from your favorite local BBQ joint.

- Portable Lunches for Work or School

Here are some ideas for portable lunches that are perfect for work or school:
1. Sandwiches: Classics like turkey, ham, or PB&J are easy to make and pack.
2. Wraps: Tortilla wraps with chicken, tuna, or veggies are a great option.
3. Salads: Pack a small container of greens and add protein like chicken, tuna, or tofu.

4. Fruits and Veggies: Carrot sticks, apple slices, and grapes are easy to pack and healthy.

5. Leftovers: Use last night's dinner as a packable lunch by reheating it in the morning.

6. Soup: Pack a thermos of soup, like tomato or black bean, with a side of crackers.

7. Bento Box: Pack a variety of small dishes like edamame, hard-boiled eggs, and crackers.

8. Quesadillas: Fill tortillas with cheese, beans, and veggies for a satisfying lunch.

9. Mini Quiches: Whip up a batch of mini quiches on the weekend and pack them for lunch.

10. Yogurt Parfait: Layer yogurt, granola, and fruit for a healthy and satisfying lunch.

11. Grilled Cheese: A classic grilled cheese sandwich is easy to pack and always a hit.

12. Chicken or Tuna Salad: Mix with greens and pack in a small container.

13. Mini Pitas: Fill small pitas with hummus, turkey, or veggies.

14. Rice Bowls: Pack a small container of rice and add protein like chicken or tofu.

15. Mini Muffins: Bake a batch of mini muffins on the weekend and pack them for lunch.

Remember to pack plenty of water or a refillable water bottle to stay hydrated!

Chapter 6:

Flavorful Dinner Recipes

Here are some flavorful dinner recipes for you to try

- Spicy Shrimp Tacos with Garlic Cilantro Lime Slaw: This dish is packed with avocado, spicy shrimp, and a homemade creamy lime slaw.
- Creamy Garlic Sun-Dried Tomato Pasta: This dish is filled with garlicky spirali noodles and tender sun-dried tomatoes in a creamy, luscious sauce with a heavy dusting of Parmesan cheese.
- Creamy Thai Sweet Potato Curry: This curry is packed with nutrition and is an easy, healthy, winter comfort food recipe.
- Red Curry Noodles: This dish has fresh veggies, seared tofu, slurpable noodles, and a saucy coconut red curry sauce.
- Instant Pot Coconut Tandoori-Inspired Chicken: This dish is made with rich spices and creamy coconut milk.
- Couscous Summer Salad: This salad is made with spiced couscous, juicy nectarines, crunchy cucumber, avocado, chickpeas, cherries, sweet corn, and mint.
- Instant Pot Chicken Cacciatore: This dish is braised Italian chicken in saucy pasta-friendly form that is bright, acidic, rich, and savory.

- CrunchyRoll Bowls: This dish is made with a block of tofu, nicely browned in teriyaki sauce, served on a bed of sticky rice with edamame, cucumber, avocado, jalapeño, and a heaping tablespoon of finely chopped, crispy onions, all covered in a generous layer of additional teriyaki and hot mayonnaise.
- BBQ Salmon Bowls with Mango Avocado Salsa: This dish is an easy and impressive dinner with yummy smoky-sweet flavor and a zip of zesty homemade salsa.
- Harissa Chickpeas with Whipped Feta: This dish is made with perfectly spicy/saucy/tomato-y chickpeas smothered in creamy, garlicky whipped feta and served with naan, lemons, and cucumbers.
- Pineapple Pork with Coconut Rice: This dish is made with sticky-sweet pork, juicy pineapple, fresh herbs, jalapeño, and crispy onions all served over a bed of fluffy coconut rice.
- Mediterranean Cod en Papillote: This dish is made with flaky baked cod and perfectly steamed veggies infused with fresh Mediterranean flavors.
- Chicken Stir-Fry: A quick supper that the whole family will enjoy, this 30-minute dish is full of bright vegetables and succulent chicken.
- Shrimp Scampi: This classic dish is cooked in the most fragrant garlic butter sauce. Yes, making it only takes ten minutes or so.
- Best Baked Chicken: This dish is made with juicy and tender chicken

breasts with this foolproof baked chicken that takes only 25 minutes.
- Mediterranean Ground Beef Stir Fry: This easy stir fry dinner is very customizable and tastes great served with rice, lentils, and more.
- Tuna Salad: This creamy and crunchy tuna salad always ticks the box.Moreover, it goes well with lettuce wraps or toast.
- Best Baked Salmon: This easy 15-minute dinner achieves perfectly tender salmon coated in lemon garlic butter and fresh herbs.
- Turkey Burgers: These turkey patties can be made in under 30 minutes and they're super juicy.
- Asian Chicken Lettuce Wraps: This 30-minute dish is ideal for a flavorful and light option. Made with chicken lettuce!

- Wholesome Dinners the Whole Family Will Love

Here are some wholesome dinner ideas that your whole family will love [1]:
- Halloumi Wraps: a simple wrap with halloumi cheese, red pesto, avocado, and walnuts.
- Lemon Ricotta Pasta: a simple and quick pasta dish.
- Air Fryer Chicken Cutlets: a quick and easy dinner with crispy and juicy chicken.
- Creamy Pesto Pasta: a quick and comforting pasta dish with vibrant and garlicky pesto sauce.

- Air Fryer Meatballs: easy to make and juicy meatballs.
- Instant Pot Bolognese: a quick and hearty pasta sauce.
- Grilled Fish Tacos with Mango Salsa: a match made in heaven with grilled flaky white fish and sweet and spicy mango salsa.
- Marry Me Chicken Pasta: a creamy and flavorful pasta dish.
- Baked Chicken Tenders: healthier and delicious baked chicken tenders.
- Garlic Butter Shrimp Pasta: a delicious combination of tender shrimp, al dente pasta, and flavorful garlic butter sauce.
- Spanish Chicken Stew: a quick and flavorful chicken stew.
- Easy Pesto Pasta: a delicious and easy summer dinner.
- Air Fryer Steak Bites: a quick and flavorful steak bites.
- Spinach Lemon Orzo: a creamy and flavorful one-pan dinner.
- Easy Paella: a classic and easy paella recipe.
- Roasted Cherry Tomato Pasta: a flavorful and easy-to-prepare pasta dish.
- Lemon Pepper Salmon: a delicious and easy salmon recipe.
- French Bread Pizza: a crispy and cheesy pizza.
- Cheesy Tortellini Casserole: a comforting and delicious casserole.
- Crispy Oven BBQ Chicken: a crispy and flavorful BBQ chicken recipe.

- One-Pot Meals for Easy Cleanup

Here are some one-pot meals that are easy to clean up [1]:
- Chicken in a Pot: a simple dish with complex flavors
- Italian Chicken Skillet: chicken, tomatoes, fresh spinach, and mozzarella
- Lemon Parmesan Chicken and Rice Bowl: cheesy, lemony, and crunchy
- Addictive Asian Beef Slaw: beef and slaw in a skillet
- Quinoa Chicken: easy to make, healthy, high protein
- Singapore Noodle Curry Shrimp: shrimp curry made with one skillet
- Spicy Unstuffed Cabbage: cabbage casserole with beef
- Gyudon Japanese Beef Bowl: beef and caramelized onions on top of short-grain rice
- One Pan Orecchiette Pasta: orecchiette pasta recipe with a handful of ingredients
- Ranch-Baked Chicken Thighs with Bacon, Brussels Sprouts, and Potatoes: chicken thighs with Brussels sprouts, potatoes, and bacon all in one pan
- One Skillet Mexican Quinoa: quinoa with shrimp, lime, and garlic
- Chicken Escabeche: chicken breasts, onions, and carrots stew in vinegar and wine
- Turkey Spaghetti Zoodles: spaghetti with turkey

- One-Pot Ham and Veggie Pasta: farfalle pasta with ham, onions, peas, and carrots
- Easy One-Pan Chicken Fried Rice: fried rice with leftover chicken and rice
- One-Pot Mediterranean Chicken: chicken with Mediterranean spices
- Arroz Con Pollo (Chicken and Rice): chicken and rice with Latin American influences
- Italian Sausage, Peppers, and Onions: sausage and peppers recipe

- International Flavors Made Diabetes-Friendly

Here are some international flavors made diabetes-friendly:

1. _Kung Pao Chicken_: Stir-fry chicken, peanuts, veggies, and brown rice for a Chinese-inspired dish.

2. _Indian Butter Chicken_: Marinate chicken in yogurt and spices, serve with brown rice and veggies.

3. _Mexican Chiles Rellenos_: Stuff bell peppers with cheese, beans, and veggies, bake until tender.

4. _Thai Green Curry_: Cook green curry paste with coconut milk, veggies, and brown rice.

5. _Japanese Teriyaki Salmon_: Grill salmon with a sweet and savory teriyaki sauce, serve with brown rice and steamed veggies.

6. _Moroccan Chickpea Tagine_: Stew chickpeas, veggies, and spices in a flavorful tomato sauce, serve with brown rice or whole wheat bread.

7. _Korean Bibimbap_: Mix rice, veggies, and protein (like beef or tofu) in a bowl, topped with a fried egg.

8. _Middle Eastern Falafel_: Crispy chickpea patties served in a pita with veggies and tzatziki sauce.

9. _Chinese Vegetable Stir-Fry_: Stir-fry a variety of colorful veggies with brown rice and a small amount of oil.

10. _Indian Vegetable Korma_: Cook veggies in a creamy tomato sauce with brown rice and naan bread.

These dishes are modified to be diabetes-friendly by:

- Snacking on brown rice rather than white rice
- Selecting lean protein sources such as tofu, fish, and poultry
- Incorporating plenty of veggies and fiber-rich ingredients
- Limiting added sugars and using natural sweeteners like yogurt and tomatoes
- Flavoring food using herbs and spices rather than sugar and salt

Note: Consult with a healthcare professional or registered dietitian for personalized dietary advice.

- Comfort Food Classics Remade for Health

Here are some comfort food classics remade for health:

1. _Mac and Cheese_: Made with whole wheat pasta, low-fat cheese, and added veggies like steamed broccoli.

2. _Chicken Pot Pie_: Made with whole wheat crust, lean chicken, and added veggies like carrots and peas.

3. _Meatloaf_: Made with lean ground turkey, whole wheat breadcrumbs, and added veggies like onions and bell peppers.

4. _Mashed Potatoes_: Made with sweet potatoes, low-fat milk, and added garlic and herbs for flavor.

5. _Fried Chicken_: Made with baked chicken, whole wheat breadcrumbs, and added spices for flavor.

6. _Grilled Cheese Sandwich_: Made with whole wheat bread, low-fat cheese, and added tomato and spinach for added nutrition.

7. _Beef Stew_: Made with lean beef, whole wheat bread, and added veggies like carrots and potatoes.

8. _Baked Apple Pie_: Made with whole wheat crust, low-fat sugar, and added cinnamon and nutmeg for flavor.

9. _Creamy Tomato Soup_: Made with low-fat cream, whole wheat crackers, and added veggies like celery and carrots.

10. _Breakfast Pancakes_: Made with whole wheat flour, low-fat milk, and added fruit like blueberries and bananas.

These comfort food classics have been remade with healthier ingredients and cooking methods to make them more nutritious and guilt-free. Enjoy!

Chapter 7:

Irresistible Snack and Dessert Recipes

Here are some irresistible snack and dessert recipes
- Jam-Topped Mini Cheesecakes: Bite-sized cheesecakes with a dollop of your favorite jam.
- Dark Chocolate Hummus: A sweet and healthy dessert hummus made with dark chocolate.
- Strawberry Cheesecake Bites: Bite-sized cheesecakes filled with strawberry and cream cheese.
- Caramel Delight Energy Balls: No-bake energy balls made with caramel, dark chocolate, and oats.
- Mini Frozen Yogurt Parfaits: Bite-sized parfaits made with frozen yogurt, fruit, and granola.
- S'mores Energy Balls: No-bake energy balls made with chocolate, marshmallows, and graham crackers.
- Raspberry Coconut Yogurt Bark: A healthy and colorful dessert made with yogurt, raspberries, and coconut.
- Mini Chocolate Chip Sandwich Cookies: Bite-sized cookies filled with chocolate chips.
- Orange-Nutella Cookie Cups: Bite-sized cookies filled with Nutella and orange zest.
- Finger-Licking Good Mini Cream Puffs: Bite-sized cream puffs filled with whipped cream and chocolate.

- Healthy Snack Options to Keep Hunger at Bay

Here are some healthy snack options to keep hunger at bay

- Edamame: Steamed soybeans are a tasty and filling snack.
- Tortilla Pinwheels: These cheesy pinwheels are easy to make and can be stored for days.
- Nutty Apple Butter: A creamy riff on a classic peanut butter and jelly sandwich.
- Crisp Cucumber Salsa: A crunchy and fresh snack.
- Stuffed Asiago-Basil Mushrooms: A healthy and savory snack.
- Carrot Cookie Bites: Soft and delicious cookies that are perfect for a snack.
- Caprese Salad Kabobs: A colorful and healthy snack.
- Mixed Berry Sundaes: A healthy and delicious dessert or snack.
- Spicy Watermelon Salsa: A vibrant and flavorful snack.
- Mediterranean Eggplant Dip: A healthy and tasty dip.
- Spicy Almonds: A healthy and flavorful snack.
- Asparagus with Fresh Basil Sauce: A tasty and healthy dip or sandwich spread.
- Pickled Brussels Sprouts: A tasty and crunchy snack.
- Chunky Blue Cheese Dip: A delicious and healthy dip.

- Rosemary Walnuts: A tasty and healthy snack.
- Homemade Guacamole: A healthy and tasty dip.
- Marinated Mozzarella: A tasty and healthy snack.
- Cinnamon Granola Bars: A healthy and tasty snack.
- Pastrami Roll-Ups: A tasty and healthy snack.
- Chocolate-Hazelnut Fruit Pizza: A tasty and healthy snack.
- Rosemary-Parmesan Popcorn: A tasty and healthy snack.
- Roasted Vegetable Dip: A tasty and healthy dip.
- Cucumber-Stuffed Cherry Tomatoes: A tasty and healthy snack.
- Peanut Butter, Honey & Pear Open-Faced Sandwiches: A tasty and healthy snack.
- Nuts: Nuts are an excellent source of fiber, protein, and good fats.
- Greek Yogurt with Berries: A tasty and healthy snack that is high in protein.
- Apple with Peanut Butter: A tasty and healthy snack that is high in fiber and protein.
- Cottage Cheese with Fruit: A tasty and healthy snack that is high in protein.
- Celery Sticks with Cream Cheese: A tasty and healthy snack that is low in carbs.
- Kale Chips with Olive Oil: A tasty and healthy snack that is high in fiber and antioxidants.

- Dark Chocolate and Almonds: A tasty and healthy snack that is high in antioxidants and healthy fats.
- Cucumber with Hummus: A tasty and healthy snack that is high in fiber and protein.
- Fruit: A tasty and healthy snack that is high in fiber and minerals.
- Tomatoes with Mozzarella Cheese: A tasty and healthy snack that is high in protein and fiber.
- Chia Seeds: A tasty and healthy snack that is high in fiber and protein.
- Eggs: A tasty and healthy snack that is high in protein.
- *Carrots with Blue Cheese Dressing*: A tasty and healthy snack that is high in fiber and protein.
- Cheese: A tasty and healthy snack that is high in protein and calcium.
- Beef Jerky: A tasty and healthy snack that is high in protein.
- Protein Smoothie: A tasty and healthy snack that is high in protein.
- Canned Fish: A tasty and healthy snack that is high in omega-3 fatty acids.
- Edamame: A tasty and healthy snack that is high in protein and fiber.
- Oats: A tasty and healthy snack that is high in fiber and protein.
- Pear Slices with Ricotta Cheese: A tasty and healthy snack that is high in fiber and protein.
- Trail Mix: A tasty and healthy snack that is high in fiber, protein and healthy fats.
- Turkey Roll-Ups: A tasty and healthy snack that is high in protein.

- Olives: A tasty and healthy snack that is high in healthy fats and antioxidants.
- Avocado: A tasty and healthy snack that is high in fiber and healthy fats.
- Air-Popped Popcorn: A tasty and healthy snack that is high in fiber.
- Roasted Chickpeas: A tasty and healthy snack that is high in fiber and protein.
- Cantaloupe: A tasty and healthy snack that is high in fiber and vitamins A and C.

- Sweet Treats Without Spiking Blood Sugar

Here are some sweet treats that don't spike blood sugar
- Dark Chocolate: Rich in flavonoids, which help prevent insulin resistance and protect against heart problems. Opt for dark chocolate with at least 70% cocoa content.
- Fresh Fruits: Fruits like pears, apples, and grapes are rich in fiber, which slows down sugar absorption in the bloodstream.
- Greek Yogurt: Rich in protein, which helps control appetite and decrease cravings for unhealthy snacks.
- *Chia Pudding*: Made with chia seeds, almond milk, and honey, this dessert is rich in fiber, protein, and omega-3 fatty acids.
- Low-Carb Energy Bites: Made with nuts, seeds, and dates, these energy balls are rich in fiber and protein.

- Cottage Cheese Fruit Bowl: A combination of cottage cheese and fruits provides protein and fiber.
- Trail Mix: A mix of nuts and seeds is rich in protein and fiber.
- Protein Smoothie: A blend of milk, protein powder, leafy greens, and fruits provides fiber and protein.
- Keto Chocolate Cake: Made with sugar-free sweeteners, this cake is low in carbs and added sugar.
- Black Bean Brownies: Made with unsweetened applesauce, dates, and black beans, these brownies are rich in fiber and protein.
- Almond Flour Caramel Cake: Made with almond flour, unsweetened almond milk, and dates, this cake is low in carbs and added sugar.
- Vegan Chocolate Avocado Mousse: Made with avocados, this mousse is rich in healthy fats and fiber.
- Keto Peanut Butter Cookies: Made with peanut butter, eggs, and monk fruit, these cookies are sugar-free and low in carbs.
- Sweetener-Free Raspberry Chia Pudding: Made with coconut milk, chia seeds, and raspberries, this pudding is rich in fiber and healthy fats.

- Guilt-Free Desserts for Special Occasions

Here are some guilt-free desserts for special occasions

- Air Fryer Churros: A healthier alternative to traditional churros using an air fryer.
- Vegan Apple Cake: A moist and flavorful cake made with eight simple ingredients.
- Air-Fryer Chocolate Chip Oatmeal Cookies: A healthier take on the classic chocolate chip cookie.
- Vegan Lemon Tart: A delicious and easy-to-make lemon tart with a flaky and creamy filling.
- Air Fryer Brownies: A healthier take on the classic brownie.
- Vegan Tiramisu: A light and airy dessert made with homemade egg-free ladyfingers.
- Air Baked Molten Lava Cake: A healthier take on the classic molten lava cake.
- Vegan Custard: A smooth and creamy custard made with five simple ingredients.
- Air Fryer Donuts: A healthier take on the classic donut.
- Vegan Cheesecake: A creamy and delicious cheesecake made without nuts, blending, or cooking.

- Smart Swaps for Your Favorite Snacks and Sweets

Here are some healthy alternatives for your favorite snacks and sweets
- Dark Chocolate: Dark chocolate with 70% or higher cacao content is a healthier alternative to regular chocolate.

- Cacao Nibs: Instead of chocolate chips, use cacao nibs for baking or as a topping.
- Banana "Nice" Cream: Freeze bananas and blend them for a healthier ice cream alternative.
- Greek Yogurt: Replace sour cream with Greek yogurt for more protein and probiotics.
- Dates and Honey: Instead of refined sugar, use dates and honey for a sweetener.
- Veggie Sticks with Hummus: Crunch on veggie sticks with hummus instead of chips.
- Farro: Replace pasta with farro for a fiber and protein-rich alternative.
- Seltzer Water: Instead of diet soda, drink seltzer water for a healthier alternative.
- Open-Face Sandwich: Use only one slice of bread for a healthier sandwich alternative.
- Chia Seed Pudding: Instead of pudding, eat chia seed pudding for a protein and fiber-rich snack.

Chapter 8:

Meal Plans and Sample Menus

Here are some meal plans and sample menus:
Meal Plans:
1. Healthy Balanced Meal Plan: A balanced meal plan with protein,

healthy fats, and complex carbohydrates.

2. Vegan Meal Plan: A plant-based meal plan with vegan alternatives to dairy and meat.

3. Gluten-Free Meal Plan: A meal plan that excludes gluten-containing ingredients.

4. Low-Carb Meal Plan: A meal plan that restricts carbohydrate intake.

5. Keto Meal Plan: A high-fat, low-carbohydrate meal plan.

Sample Menus:

Breakfast

- Healthy Balanced Meal Plan: Oatmeal with fruit and nuts

- Vegan Meal Plan: Tofu scramble with vegetables and whole grain toast

- Gluten-Free Meal Plan: Gluten-free pancakes with fresh berries

- Low-Carb Meal Plan: Scrambled eggs with spinach and avocado

- Keto Meal Plan: Keto coffee with coconut oil and heavy cream

Lunch

- Healthy Balanced Meal Plan: Grilled chicken salad with mixed greens and whole grain crackers

- Vegan Meal Plan: Lentil soup with whole grain bread

- Gluten-Free Meal Plan: Grilled chicken breast with roasted vegetables and quinoa

- Low-Carb Meal Plan: Turkey lettuce wraps with avocado and tomato

- Keto Meal Plan: Keto Cobb salad with grilled chicken and avocado

Dinner

- Healthy Balanced Meal Plan: Grilled salmon with roasted vegetables and brown rice
- Vegan Meal Plan: Vegan stir-fry with tofu and brown rice
- Gluten-Free Meal Plan: Grilled chicken breast with roasted sweet potatoes and green beans
- Low-Carb Meal Plan: Grilled steak with roasted broccoli and cauliflower
- Keto Meal Plan: Keto beef stir-fry with vegetables and cauliflower rice

Snacks

- Healthy Balanced Meal Plan: Fresh fruit and nuts
- Vegan Meal Plan: Vegan energy balls with oats and nuts
- Gluten-Free Meal Plan: Gluten-free crackers with hummus
- Low-Carb Meal Plan: Cheese and vegetables
- Keto Meal Plan: Keto fat bombs with coconut oil and chocolate
- Weekly Meal Plans for Balanced Nutrition

Here is a 7-day meal plan for balanced nutrition

Day 1

- Breakfast: Smoked salmon and egg on a whole grain bagel with watercress and a low-fat mocha drink
- Lunch: Bean and vegetable soup with whole grain seeded bread and a side of steamed vegetables and fruit
- Dinner: Greek mac and cheese casserole with steamed broccoli and Greek yogurt with berries and nuts for dessert

Day 2

- Breakfast: Berry smoothie with protein powder
- Lunch: Tuna salad sandwich on whole grain bread with root vegetable chips and sliced crudités and a banana
- Dinner: Salmon with pineapple-avocado salsa and leafy greens, followed by cocoa chia seed pudding with strawberries and an oat milk hot drink

Day 3

- Breakfast: Oatmeal with banana, pumpkin seeds, and maple syrup, coffee with low-fat milk
- Lunch: Mashed avocado, roast turkey, and chopped tomatoes on whole grain toast with extra virgin olive oil, shelled hemp seeds, and cayenne pepper, with a side of blueberries
- Dinner: Chicken and vegetable stir-fry served with steamed brown rice, dark chocolate, and walnuts

Day 4

- Breakfast: Apple and peanut butter on a whole wheat English muffin with low-fat milk
- Lunch: Baked potato with beef chili and creme fraiche, with a side of green beans or peas
- Dinner: Veggie Korean bibimbap with kombucha drink

Day 5

- Breakfast: Granola, Greek yogurt, blueberries, flax seeds, and coffee with low-fat milk
- Lunch: Tuna salad sandwich on whole grain bread with salad

vegetables, a banana, nuts, an orange, and lemon and ginger herbal tea
- Dinner: Rotisserie chicken tacos with pineapple salsa, baked sweet potato, arugula, dark chocolate, and walnuts
Day 6
- Breakfast: Quinoa edamame egg muffins with grilled tomatoes and mushrooms, almond milk
- Lunch: Slow cooker black bean soup with watercress and roasted squash with paprika and rosemary
- Dinner: Baked potato with chili, creme fraiche, leafy greens, dark chocolate, and walnuts
Day 7
- Breakfast: Sardines on whole grain toast with spread, fresh spinach, and low-fat mocha drink
- Lunch: Grilled chicken fillet with broccoli, carrots, corn on the cob, and an orange
- Dinner: Slow cooker sweet potato curry with cauliflower rice, wheat paratha, and satsuma, with a kombucha drink

- Sample Menus for Different Caloric Needs

Here are some sample menus for different caloric needs:
1200 Calories
- Oatmeal with fruit and nuts for breakfast (300 calories)
- Snack: Carrot sticks with hummus (100 calories)

- Lunch: Grilled chicken salad with mixed greens and whole grain crackers (400 calories)
- Snack: 150-calorie slices of apple with almond butter
- Dinner: Baked salmon with roasted vegetables and quinoa (350 calories)

1500 Calories

- Breakfast: Greek yogurt with berries and granola (400 calories)
- Snack: Hard-boiled egg and cherry tomatoes (120 calories)
- Lunch: Turkey and avocado wrap with mixed greens and whole grain tortilla (500 calories)
- Snack: Rice cakes with peanut butter and banana slices (180 calories)
- Dinner: Grilled chicken breast with roasted sweet potatoes and green beans (400 calories)

1800 Calories

- Breakfast: Smoothie bowl with protein powder, banana, spinach, and almond milk (500 calories)
- Snack: Cottage cheese with cucumber slices and whole grain crackers (150 calories)
- Lunch: Grilled chicken and quinoa bowl with roasted vegetables and avocado (600 calories)
- Snack: Apple slices with cheddar cheese (170 calories)
- Dinner: Baked chicken thighs with roasted broccoli and brown rice (550 calories)

2000 Calories

- Breakfast: Avocado toast with scrambled eggs and whole grain bread (550 calories)

- Snack: Greek yogurt with honey and mixed nuts (200 calories)
- Lunch: Grilled chicken and vegetable stir-fry with brown rice (700 calories)
- Snack: Protein bar (200 calories)
- Dinner: Grilled salmon with roasted asparagus and quinoa (600 calories)

2500 Calories

- Breakfast: Breakfast burrito with scrambled eggs, black beans, and avocado (700 calories)
- Snack: Apple slices with peanut butter and banana slices (250 calories)
- Lunch: Turkey and cheese sandwich on whole grain bread with carrot sticks and hummus (800 calories)
- Snack: Protein smoothie with banana, spinach, and almond milk (300 calories)
- Dinner: Grilled chicken and vegetable kebabs with quinoa and pita bread (800 calories)

Note: These menus are just examples and may need to be adjusted based on individual calorie needs and dietary preferences. It's always best to consult with a healthcare professional or registered dietitian for personalized nutrition recommendations.

- Adjusting Meal Plans for Varied Dietary Preferences

Here's how to adjust meal plans for varied dietary preferences:
Vegetarian/Vegan:
- Replace meat with plant-based protein sources like beans, lentils, tofu, and tempeh.

- Use veggie broth rather than beef or chicken broth.
- Choose vegan-friendly milk alternatives like almond milk, soy milk, or coconut milk.

Gluten-Free:
- Replace wheat bread with gluten-free bread or whole grain gluten-free options.
- Choose gluten-free grains like quinoa, brown rice, and corn.
- Be mindful of hidden sources of gluten in sauces and seasonings.

Low-Carb:
- Reduce or eliminate high-carb foods like bread, pasta, and sugary snacks.
- Increase protein and healthy fat intake.
- Choose low-carb vegetables like leafy greens, broccoli, and cauliflower.

Keto:
- Significantly reduce carbohydrate intake.
- Increase fat intake with healthy fats like avocado, nuts, and olive oil.
- Moderate protein intake.

Low-Fat/Low-Sodium:
- Opt for lean protein sources such as tofu, fish, and chicken.
- Limit added fats like oil, butter, and cream.
- Use herbs and spices rather than salt for seasoning.

Halal/Kosher:
- Follow Islamic or Jewish dietary laws.
- Choose halal or kosher-certified meat and poultry.
- Avoid pork and pork products.

Raw Food:
- Incorporate more raw fruits and vegetables.
- Use raw nuts and seeds as snacks.
- Choose raw milk and cheese alternatives.
Remember to consult with a healthcare professional or registered dietitian for personalized nutrition recommendations.

Chapter 9:

Lifestyle Tips for Long-Term Diabetes Wellness

Here are some lifestyle tips for long-term diabetes wellness:

1. Healthy Eating: Focus on whole, unprocessed foods like vegetables, fruits, whole grains, lean proteins, and healthy fats. Aim for a balanced diet that is low in added sugars, salt, and saturated fats.

2. Physical Activity: Engage in regular physical activity, such as walking, swimming, or other aerobic exercises, for at least 150 minutes per week. This can help manage blood sugar levels and improve overall health.

3. Weight Management: Maintain a healthy weight through a combination of healthy eating and regular physical activity. This can enhance general health and lower the chance of issues.

4. Stress Management: Engage in stress-reducing activities like yoga,

meditation, or deep breathing exercises to help manage stress and anxiety.

5. Sleep: Aim for 7-8 hours of sleep per night to help regulate blood sugar levels and improve overall health.

6. Stay Hydrated: Drink plenty of water throughout the day to help regulate blood sugar levels and prevent dehydration.

7. Monitor Blood Sugar: Regularly monitor blood sugar levels to understand how different foods, activities, and stress levels affect your levels.

8. Medication Adherence: Take medications as prescribed by your healthcare provider to help manage blood sugar levels and prevent complications.

9. Regular Check-Ups: Schedule regular check-ups with your healthcare provider to monitor your condition and make any necessary adjustments to your treatment plan.

10. Support System: Build a support system of family, friends, and healthcare professionals to help you stay motivated and engaged in your diabetes management plan.

Remember, managing diabetes requires a long-term commitment to healthy lifestyle choices and regular monitoring and care. By following these tips, you can help manage your condition and improve your overall health and well-being.

- Incorporating Physical Activity into Your Routine

Incorporating physical activity into your routine can have numerous benefits for your overall health and well-being.Here are some pointers to get you going:

1. Start small: Begin with short periods of physical activity, such as 10-15 minutes a day, and gradually increase the duration and intensity over time.

2. Find activities you enjoy: Engage in physical activities that bring you joy, whether it's walking, jogging, swimming, cycling, or dancing.

3. Schedule it in: Treat physical activity as a non-negotiable part of your daily routine, just like brushing your teeth or taking a shower.

4. Find a workout buddy: Having a workout partner or accountability partner can help motivate you to stay consistent.

5. Mix it up: Vary your physical activities to avoid boredom and prevent plateaus.

6. Make it convenient: Find ways to incorporate physical activity into your daily routine, such as taking the stairs instead of the elevator or walking to work.

7. Track your progress: Use a fitness tracker, journal, or mobile app to monitor your physical activity and stay motivated.

8. Consult a healthcare professional: Before starting any new physical

activity routine, consult with a healthcare professional to discuss any health concerns or limitations.

Some examples of physical activities you can incorporate into your routine include:

- Brisk walking
- Jogging or running
- Swimming
- Cycling
- Dancing
- Yoga or Pilates
- Resistance training (weightlifting)
- High-intensity interval training (HIIT)
- Gardening or yard work
- Housework or cleaning
- Playing sports or games (e.g., tennis, basketball, soccer)

Remember, every bit counts, and even small amounts of physical activity can have significant health benefits.

- Stress Management Techniques for Better Blood Sugar Control

Here are some stress management techniques that can help with better blood sugar control:

1. _Deep Breathing Exercises_: Deep breathing can help reduce stress and anxiety, which can raise blood sugar levels.

2. _Progressive Muscle Relaxation_: This technique involves tensing and relaxing different muscle groups to release physical tension.

3. _Mindfulness Meditation_: Mindfulness meditation can help reduce stress and anxiety by focusing on the present moment.

4. _Yoga_: Yoga combines physical movement with deep breathing and meditation techniques to reduce stress and anxiety.

5. _Walking or Physical Activity_: Regular physical activity can help reduce stress and anxiety, improve mood, and lower blood sugar levels.

6. _Journaling_: Writing down your thoughts and feelings can help process and release emotions, reducing stress and anxiety.

7. _Grounding Techniques_: Grounding techniques, such as focusing on your five senses, can help bring you back to the present moment and reduce stress and anxiety.

8. _Social Support_: Connecting with friends, family, or a support group can help you feel less isolated and more supported, reducing stress and anxiety.

9. _Time Management_: Poor time management can lead to increased stress levels, so prioritize tasks, set realistic goals, and take regular breaks.

10. _Self-Care_: Make time for activities that bring you joy and relaxation, such as reading, listening to music, or taking a relaxing bath.

Remember, everyone is unique, and what works for one person may not work for another. Experiment with different techniques to find what works best for you and your blood sugar control.

- Importance of Regular Monitoring and Doctor Visits

Regular monitoring and doctor visits are crucial for effective diabetes management and overall health. Here's why:

1. Blood Sugar Control: Regular monitoring helps you understand how different foods, activities, and stress levels affect your blood sugar levels, enabling you to make informed decisions to maintain control.

2. Identifying Patterns: Monitoring helps identify patterns and trends in your blood sugar levels, allowing you to adjust your treatment plan accordingly.

3. Preventing Complications: Regular monitoring and doctor visits can help prevent or detect diabetes-related complications, such as nerve damage, kidney damage, and vision problems.

4. Medication Adjustments: Regular monitoring and doctor visits enable your healthcare provider to adjust your medication or treatment plan as needed to ensure optimal control.

5. Lifestyle Adjustments: Regular monitoring and doctor visits provide opportunities to discuss lifestyle changes, such as diet and exercise, to improve your overall health and diabetes management.

6. Early Detection of Issues: Regular monitoring and doctor visits can detect potential issues, such as hypoglycemia

(low blood sugar) or hyperglycemia (high blood sugar), allowing for prompt treatment.

7. Improved Quality of Life: Regular monitoring and doctor visits can help you feel more in control of your diabetes, reducing stress and anxiety and improving your overall quality of life.

8. Reduced Risk of Long-term Complications: Regular monitoring and doctor visits can help reduce the risk of long-term complications, such as heart disease, stroke, and kidney disease.

Remember, regular monitoring and doctor visits are essential for effective diabetes management and overall health. Stay committed to your monitoring schedule and doctor visits to ensure optimal control and improved quality of life.

- Building a Support System for Diabetes Management

Building a support system is crucial for effective diabetes management. Here are a few strategies for creating a solid support network:

1. _Family and Friends_: Educate them about diabetes and its management. Encourage them to enquire and provide assistance.

2. _Diabetes Support Group_: Join a local support group or online community to connect with others who understand your challenges.

3. _Healthcare Team_: Build a relationship with your healthcare provider, nurse, and other specialists. Ask questions and seek guidance.

4. _Mental Health Professional_: Consider seeking help from a therapist or counselor to cope with emotional challenges.

5. _Online Resources_: Utilize reputable websites, apps, and online forums for education, support, and connection.

6. _Peer Support_: Connect with others who have diabetes through organizations like the American Diabetes Association.

7. _Caregiver Support_: If you have a caregiver, ensure they receive support and education as well.

8. _Diabetes Educator_: Work with a certified diabetes educator for personalized guidance and support.

Remember, a strong support system can help you stay motivated, informed, and empowered to manage your diabetes effectively.Reach out and expand your network of supporters without fear!

Conclusion

In conclusion, managing diabetes requires a comprehensive approach that incorporates healthy lifestyle choices, regular monitoring, and a strong support system. By following the tips and strategies outlined in this guide, you can effectively manage your diabetes and improve your overall health and well-being.

Remember, diabetes management is a journey, and it's essential to be patient, persistent, and kind to yourself along the way. Don't hesitate to seek help when you need it, and celebrate your successes, no matter how small they may seem.

With the right mindset and tools, you can thrive with diabetes and live a long, healthy, and fulfilling life. Keep in mind that knowledge is power, and staying informed about the latest developments in diabetes management will help you make informed decisions about your care.

Stay positive, stay proactive, and remember that you are not alone in your diabetes journey. There are many resources available to support you, and with time and effort, you can achieve optimal diabetes management and live a life that is full, rich, and rewarding.

- Embracing Your Journey to Diabetes Wellness

Embracing your journey to diabetes wellness requires a mindset shift from merely managing your condition to actively taking control of your health and well-being. Here are some key aspects to embrace:

1. Acceptance: Acknowledge your diabetes diagnosis and understand that it's a part of your life.

2. Empowerment: Take ownership of your health and wellness journey, making informed decisions and seeking support when needed.

3. Self-care: Prioritize your physical, emotional, and mental well-being, recognizing that self-care is essential for overall health.

4. Education: Stay informed about diabetes management, new technologies, and research advancements to make informed decisions.

5. Resilience: Develop coping strategies to navigate challenges and setbacks, focusing on progress rather than perfection.

6. Support network: Surround yourself with understanding family, friends, and healthcare professionals who encourage and support your journey.

7. Holistic approach: Address your physical, emotional, and mental health by incorporating healthy habits, stress management, and mindfulness practices.

8. Celebrating milestones: Acknowledge and celebrate your achievements, no matter how small, to stay motivated and encouraged.

9. Self-compassion: Be kind, patient, and understanding to yourself as you would a close friend.

10. Hope and optimism: Maintain a positive outlook, focusing on the possibilities and opportunities for a healthy, fulfilling life with diabetes.

By embracing these aspects, you'll transform your journey to diabetes wellness into a empowering and transformative experience that enriches your life.

- **Final Words of Encouragement and Inspiration**

Remember, managing diabetes is a journey, not a destination. It's okay to take it one day at a time, to learn as you go, and to ask for help when you need it. You are stronger than you think, and you are capable of achieving great things.

Don't let diabetes define you - you are so much more than your diagnosis. You are a unique, talented, and valuable person with so much to offer the world.

Keep pushing forward, even when it's hard. Celebrate your small wins, and don't be too proud to ask for help when you need it. You are not alone in this journey - there are countless others who understand what you're going through, and who are cheering you on every step of the way.

Remember to be kind to yourself, to take care of your body and mind, and to never give up hope. You got this!

And always remember: you are more than your diabetes. You are a warrior, a fighter, and a survivor. Keep shining your light, and never let your diagnosis hold you back from living the life you deserve.

1 total reaction